YO[illegible] BASICS

A Beginner's Guide To Attaining Inner Peace, Living A Stress-Free Life And Achieving Your Weight Goals

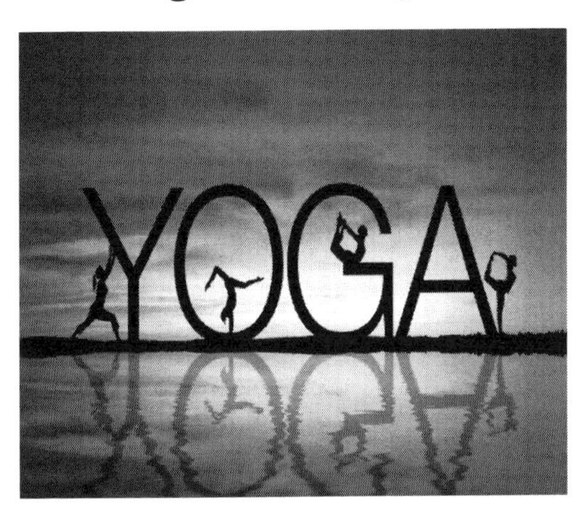

By

Fhilcar Faunillan

Table of Contents

INTRODUCTION

I want to thank you and congratulate you for downloading the book, *"Yoga Basics: A Beginner's Guide to Attaining Inner Peace, Living a Stress-Free Life and Achieving Your Weight Goals."*

Yoga is a term you hear almost everywhere. Whether as a form of exercise or purely for meditation, a lot have embraced this.

In this book, you will learn the basic information you need to know about yoga. This book will guide you as you start your practice by giving you the list of the things you need to remember and follow.

Yoga has long been known to help people achieve different goals in life such as health and wellness. It does not only improve the person's physical health, but it also helps in the development of the mind and spirit. Yoga allows a person to be closer to the self and to be a part of the universe as well. It leads a person to become fully aware and through this, it becomes easier to live a life away from stress and negative energy.

Thanks again for downloading this book, I hope you enjoy it!

Chapter 1 - What Yoga Is and What It's Not

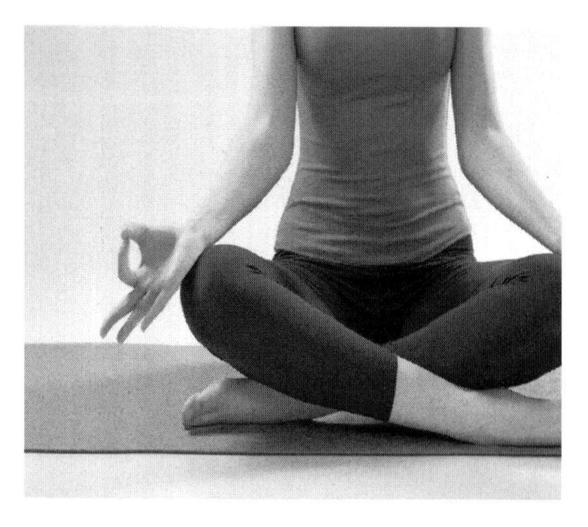

Nowadays, it is common to hear the word yoga. A lot of people are into yoga and meditation classes because they might want to lose weight or gain peace of mind. Some may even have the conception that yoga is just a form of exercise with some sort of breathing, stretching and seemingly impossible poses and twists, but yoga goes so much deeper than these things you initially thought of. However it is also important to remember that yoga cannot be easily defined in a single and diffused way since its very nature is diverse in itself.

Often times, yoga is perceived or believed to be a kind of religion but it is important to know that this is not the case. It does not come with a set of rules or beliefs and there is no certain divine god-like being to be worshipped. Anyone can practice yoga regardless of their religious affiliation or beliefs. Although many of its ideas and teaching are similar to those of Buddhism and Hinduism, yoga is neither a branch nor part of those two. This is a common misconception that needs to be refuted.

One simple definition we could give is that yoga comprises of physical, mental, and spiritual practices which aims to integrate the body, mind, and spirit to achieve a feeling of oneness with the universe. The term has been derived from the Sanskrit word 'Yuj' which means to unite the different individual aspects of the self into its original whole. Its ultimate goal is to achieve happiness that comes from the experience of being in the center of consciousness and being one with the individual's True Self. The practice of yoga can be traced back a thousand of years ago back to the times where written words were still nonexistent. During those ancient times, yoga was an intimate practice between a yoga master and his disciple.

The foundations of the ancient yoga system are generally linked to the Patanjali, a great Indian sage, who summarized the approach of the Yoga Sutra. Throughout the past centuries, the meaning of yoga has shifted and the approaches to Yoga have developed.

At present, yoga instructors will often refer to your practice as an individual experience that develops over a period of time. Over time, the practice of yoga is constantly changing and evolving so it never gets boring. The poses might not necessarily change from time to time but your attitude and relationship towards the practice itself definitely will.

Majority of Western ideas about yoga have influenced people to associate it with only the physical aspect of yoga which includes the physical asana and breathing practice. Again, as implied earlier, there is more to yoga than defining it as a mere physical practice. In reality, this physical aspect of yoga, which is called Hatha Yoga, is only one of its many branches or paths. Aside from Hatha, the other five main branches include Karma, Jnana, Raja, Tantra, and Bhakti.

1. **Hatha Yoga or the Yoga of Postures**

   This is perhaps the most popular and familiar branch of yoga in the West. This refers to the physical path or the Yoga of Postures. Hatha Yoga sees the human body as the carrier for the soul that is why it seeks to bring in perfect health through physical asana, meditation, and breathing techniques. The goal of the Hatha Yoga practice is to unite the soul to the body and make sure the union is in a perfect condition. Within this Path of Yoga, there are different styles of practice which includes Iyengar, Jiva Mukti, Integral, among others.

2. **Bhakti Yoga or the Yoga of Devotion**

   This branch of Yoga is the path of the heart and devotion to a higher power or being. Bhakti Yoga is the most followed path in India. It involves a person's relationship with his beliefs that is why the experience might be different for each one. Those who follow this path try to see the good in everything and everyone. This allows a person to love, tolerate, and accept the things around.

3. **Jnana Yoga or the Yoga of the Mind**

This path generally focuses on the aspect of the mind and includes intelligence, contemplation, and introspection. It deals with knowledge and wisdom and then tries to unify it with a person's intellect. The Jnana path aims to allow a person to gain more knowledge and with this, it is open to all other religions and philosophies. This path holds the belief that an open, curious, and rational mind is an important key in knowing the true self.

4. **Tantra Yoga or the Yoga of Rituals**

This path of yoga is perceived to be the most misunderstood as compared to the other five. Why is that so? Because people associate it with witchcraft, spells, sorcery, and mystic aspects. It may be true that Tantra Yoga uses rituals but it does not involve any dark magic. A lot of people also view it as sexual. Although sex is a part of this path, it is not the whole picture. The Tantra yoga path only tries to find what is scared in the things we do and sex happens to be one of the basic human drive. It recognizes that there is a certain energy behind all things, whether mental or physical, and tries to honor different life aspects through rituals. A Tantra Yogi must embody humility, purity, devotion, courage, cosmic love, dedication, faithfulness, contentment, and truthfulness.

5. **Raja Yoga or the Yoga of Self-Control**

Raja Yoga is known as the royal branch as is also called Ashtanga Yoga. It involves the eight fold path or eight limbs of yoga and it focuses on contemplation and meditation. This path teaches us to honor the self because the universe exists for the self. A Raja Yogi must consider the self as the center, and with this it is important to respect the self together with all the surrounding creations vital to its unfolding. A Raji practioner must also bear in mind that in order to achieve self-respect, one must become a master of himself.

6. **Karma Yoga or the Yoga of Service**

In this path, it is believed that the things happening at present are based on your past actions. This is the reason why one must go through the path of service and

> selflessness in order to choose a future that is free from all the selfishness and negative energy. Karma Yoga teaches us that the more we do selfless acts today, the better our karma will be which is why we need to steer ourselves towards goodness - good thoughts, words, and deeds.

If you come to think of it, Yoga is not really something new to us. If you base it on the definitions of the different branches mentioned above, Yoga itself has long been present in our lives in some ways. The thing is, we were not just aware of it. As we go further, you will see how the different asana are present in the different things you do. You will also see how the principles and teachings of Yoga overlap those of your own. You will be delighted to find out that indeed, Yoga is for not only for you but everyone.

Chapter 2 - Before Getting Started

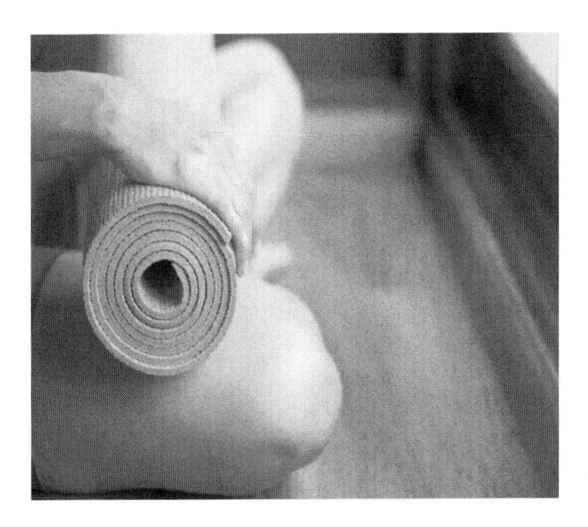

The moment you decide to start doing yoga is the first step you need. However, a lot of people get intimidated and become stuck in this phase and end up not doing any practice at all. In order to make sure that you will go on the next step of your practice, here are the things you need to know before getting started.

1. **Choose a yoga type**

There are a lot of available yoga classes out there which is why you need to be careful in choosing the ones that will fit your physical state and personality. Know your limitations. Some classes are more slow-paced and basic, while others are of a higher level. This is the part where you get to choose your own adventure because there are as many different yoga styles as there are personalities. Hatha is a classical and gentle form of yoga while Vinyasa, which is also referred to as the power yoga, is a dynamic and fluid yoga style that uses a series of asana with breathing exercises. Another style is Bikram wherein the poses are done within a heated room. Bikram yoga is quite popular nowadays and a lot of celebrities are into this type not simply to lose weight but boost confidence. For a more meditative-based yoga practice which involves a lot of chanting, Jiva Mukti yoga might work for you. If you want to focus on the alignment of your poses you can try Iyengar yoga. For starters, hatha or vinyasa class will be most appropriate and recommended.

2. Picking a class

If you are living in the metro, you will surely spot some yoga studios around your area. You might have friends who are already doing yoga classes. You can also check online sites, newspaper ads, or lifestyle magazines for classes that are convenient from where you are located. A lot of gyms also offer yoga sessions so it may be a good start especially if you are already doing gym exercises. Aside from your desire to do practice, having a good yoga teacher will help you stick to it. If you attend a class and feel that you do not click with the instructor, you can always find others. Before starting a class, try to chat with your instructor for any concern. Inform him/her that it is your first time and also mention if you have any bodily discomforts or conditions. It is important that you are comfortable with the class you are in so that it will be easier for you to go deeper into your practice.

3. **Getting your own mat**

Although some yoga studios or gym offer free use of mats during classes, it is recommended for you to bring your own. This option is more hygienic because in doing yoga, you will surely shed some sweat onto the mat. They might do some washing and drying but it is best to make sure that you don't get any skin irritations or problems from using these free mats. In addition, having your own yoga mat allows you to take your practice anywhere and anytime. If you become familiar with the routines, you can practice at home or any place of your preference. You can conveniently bring your mat by the beach and do some poses while enjoying the breeze. Here are some things you need to check on in choosing the mat that is right for you:

a. Length

When buying a mat, you need to make sure that it is long enough for your height. Make sure that your mat can fit both your hands and feet in doing poses such as Downward Dog. If you lie down during poses such as Savasana or dead man's post, try to see if your body fits the mat. Yoga mats can run up to 84 inches long.

b. Texture

In doing yoga, your mat will become one of your best friends that is why it is important to make sure that you are comfortable with the way your mat feels. Yes, that is a fact. Some mats can give the sticky feeling because of their textured grips which prevents you from slipping while performing different poses. Other mats may also have that natural texture while others are like the rubber soles.

c. Thickness and Weight

Some yoga styles may require you thicker mats so as to help you avoid getting bruised. If you practice Ashtanga, Power Yoga, or Vinyasa you might want to get a quarter-inch thick yoga mat. For more gentle and slow-paced classes, you can opt for thinner mats. The weight of the mats may also vary depending on the material and thickness so it is up to you to choose what fits you best.

4. **Gloves and Yoga Towels**

   In practicing yoga, you might end up sweating a lot more than usual because the physical aspect of yoga really works out your body. With all the sweat, it might be dangerous when the mat becomes slippery. You will be doing several poses wherein you need to balance or have a strong grip with your mat. A glove might work for some, especially those who have really sweaty hands. A good yoga mat towel may also be of use in order to soak up the sweat. There are available towels that are of perfect fit to different yoga mats. Just make sure that you pick those that dry fast and are made from extra-absorbent material.

5. **Wear the right clothes**

Practicing yoga will require you to do several poses such as stretching, balancing, among others. Remember to always wear comfortable clothes in which you can freely move your whole body. Yoga pants are available but you can also use some other clothing as long as you are comfortable wearing it. As much as possible, wear items of the right fit. Avoid those that are too big or revealing and don't wear those that are too tight as well. You don't need to get any shoes or foot wear for yoga since you will do your practice with bare feet.

6. **Have a positive mindset and be a beginner**

People become drawn to yoga because of several reasons. When you decide to begin, think of it as a chance to embrace a new life journey. Don't be afraid to be a novice and grasp the idea of a 'beginner's mind'. Go and stand on top of your mat without any notion of what poses you can or can't do. Maintain the positive mindset that the more you practice, you will gain more experience as well. Do not get intimidated with those people who can already do poses such as headstands easily. That is the reason why you need to begin, so that you will learn more about yourself and learn how to work with your body as well.

Chapter 3 - Yoga Poses

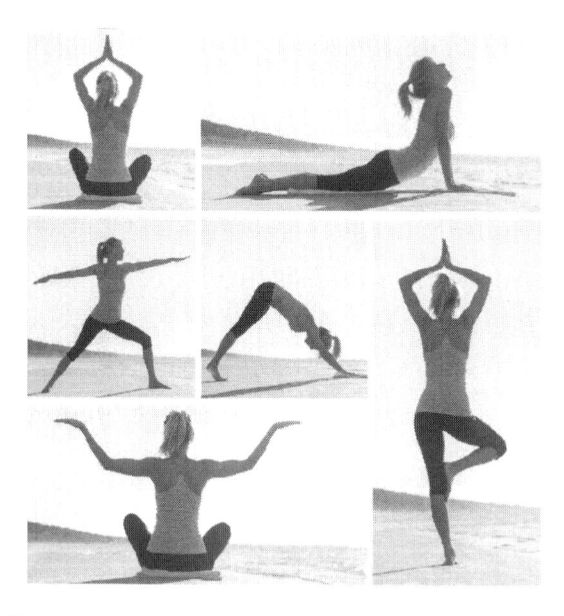

Yoga poses or asanas literally mean 'seat'. Originally, back in the ancient times, there was a single asana; the seated meditation pose. At present, there are a huge number of poses used in the practice of yoga. More than just toning, stretching, and strengthening the body, these different yoga poses open the energy and psychic channels of a person. It is a means to help purify and heal the body. Also, it allows you to calm and control your mind.

Yoga asanas can be classified in many ways depending on its usefulness, application, and levels of practice. This chapter will provide you a list of the commonly used poses in Yoga that would be helpful to you as you begin your practice. These poses are used widely in almost all styles of Yoga practice.

1. **Mountain Pose**

   This pose is the foundation or the blueprint of all standing poses. It is a good starting and resting position. Although it seems like you are just standing, this pose helps you achieve proper posture, balance, alignment, muscle strength and allows you to focus on the present moment.

   How to do it:

Stand tall and upright with your feet together or hip-width apart. Ground down and evenly distribute your weight between your feet. Then, align your hips that it should be aligned directly over your legs and feet. Lengthen your lower back, all four sides of your waist, and elongate your spine. Relax and breathe normally. Inhale and lift out of the waist, exhale and then drop your shoulders down.

2. **Chair Pose**

In this pose, you will be basically sitting in an imaginary chair. If you think about it, sitting in a chair may seem easy but this pose requires intense work and power. You really need determination in order to stay longer in this pose. This pose will help you strengthen your legs, shoulders, and back.

How to do it:

Start this position by doing the mountain pose, with your feet slightly apart. Stretch your hands in front with your palms facing downwards and try not to bend your elbows while doing so. Next thing you have to do is to bend your knees as if you were sitting in a chair. If you are already in position, try to be comfortable as possible. Also, make sure that you are keeping your hands parallel to the ground. Lengthen your spine and relax. Breathe normally and then try to go deeper into the pose by gradually going down.

3. Downward facing dog

The downward facing dog is a mix of handstand, inversion, and forward bend pose. This pose is usually done as a part of the sun salutation series but you can also it alone. It is a resting pose that is used to help you recover and catch your pace from a vigorous routine. Also, this pose helps open your shoulders and stretch your hamstring and spine. The inversion, wherein your head is positioned below your heart, creates a calming effect as well.

How to do it:

Start this pose by standing hip-width apart. Spread your toes and make sure you are in balance. While keeping your back straight, hinge forward and place your palms flat on the floor with your fingers spread apart. Bend your knees as you reach for the floor. Next, step your feet back and do a push up. Lift your hips towards the ceiling as if you are forming an inverted V. Press your chess towards your knees as far as you can and press your heels toward the floor.

4. **Upward facing dog**

The upward facing dog pose helps strengthen your shoulders, legs, wrist, arms and buttocks. This pose opens your chest and stretches out your back and shoulders. It appears after the upward facing dog in the classic sun salutation series.

How to do it:

Lie flat on your belly, stretch your body across your mat and relax. Bend your elbows and place your palms flat on the side of your chest. Try to see if your forearms are relatively perpendicular to the mat. Reach back through your legs and lift your torso up until you can straighten your arms. Next, lift your knees and thighs away from the floor and lift your breastbone up as well. Lengthen your body especially the sides and always keep your neck long. Hold the pose for several breaths and then release by going back towards your mat.

5. **Warrior Poses**

It may seem strange to associate or name a yoga pose after a warrior because yoga is about peace, happiness and not violence. Although texts of ancient yoga practice involve dialogues between warriors (i.e. Krishna and Arjuna), the warrior pose does not signify anything violent. Instead, this pose wants to show the idea of a person being a 'spiritual warrior' who fights against self-ignorance, suffering, and the evil of this world. There are three warrior poses used in the practice of yoga;

warrior 1, warrior 2, and warrior 3.

Warrior 1

This pose helps open the hips and chest. Also, it strengthens and stretches both the arms and legs. The warrior 1 pose allows you to develop balance and concentration.

How to do it:

An easy way to begin this pose is by starting with downward facing dog. Step one foot forward and position it between your hands. Turn the remaining foot at 45 degrees and make sure you have a tight ground. Align your heels together, or maybe even slightly wider. Bend your front knee over your ankle and stretch your back leg. Raise your arms up to ceiling and give your arms a stretch.

Warrior 2

The warrior 2 pose is somehow similar to that of the warrior 1. Its benefits are the same as it helps strengthen and develop the body. In addition, it also helps improve body respiration and circulation. This yoga pose energizes the whole body giving you a more positive feeling.

How to do it:

Stand with your feet wide apart with about 3 1/2 to 4 feet distance. Next is try to turn one foot in slightly and the turn the other one at 90 degrees to the side. Align your front heel with the arch of the other foot. Then, bend your front knee making a 90 degree angle and track the knee with the second toe so that your knee joint will be protected. Stretch your back leg and make sure your foot is well grounded. Reach your arms out to the sides with shoulder blades down and palms wide. Look at your front fingers and extend as far as you can.

Warrior 3

The warrior 3 pose tries to recreate the scene wherein the fierce warrior, Virabhadra, chopped off his enemy's head. This pose helps strengthen the upper back, hips, and legs. Also, it greatly improves balance and posture. For starters, balancing in this pose can be challenging but it would surely give you the satisfaction once you are able to hold it for several breaths.

How to do it:

An easy way to do this pose is by starting from warrior 1. Next step is to hinge the hips forward in a way where you can rest your abdomen on your front thigh with both your arms alongside with your ears. Shift your weight on your front foot and lift your other leg up and stretch your arms forward as if you are forming a 'T'. Hold the pose for several breaths and if you can't keep up, slowly put your back foot down and rest.

6. Triangle Pose

The triangle pose is considered one of the key standing pose in yoga. This pose helps expand and strengthen your shoulders, hips, spine and chest. It also increases mobility of body joints, specifically the hips and neck. In order to keep balance during the pose, beginners are required to open their eyes for easier execution. For those people who are not very flexible, this pose might be a challenge but as one goes deeper into practice, one can find it easier each time.

How to do it:

First thing to do is to stand feet wide apart. Next, move your right foot back, approximately 3-4 inches away from the left. Then, turn your left foot in slightly and rotate your right thigh open until your right toes become directly pointed to the side. Keep both legs straight and make sure you ground your feet properly on your mat. Pull your thighs up and spread your arms at shoulder height. After this, hinge at the front hip and touch your front ankle with one hand while you raise the other towards the ceiling, reaching as high as you can. Lengthen your spine and look up. Breathe normally and hold the pose for several seconds.

7. Revolved Triangle Pose

From the name itself, this pose is a variation of the triangle pose. Yes, it may seem hard for most but it will surely pay off as it is very helpful in opening and strengthening the hips, hamstrings, chest, back, and abdomen. It also aims to improve body circulation, digestion, and helps build attention and relieve stress.

How to do it:

This pose is similar to the triangle pose so you just have to follow the same steps for the previous pose. The difference would be that you have to rotate your body and raise your hand to the opposite side.

8. Half-moon pose

The moon is a significant symbol in yoga. Together with the sun, it represents polar energies of the body. The half-moon pose is a one-legged pose in yoga which requires a strong and stable leg. It may look easy, but it will take focus and determination to be able to do this pose. It helps strengthen your back, core, thighs, and ankles.

How to do it:

Begin the half-moon pose by doing triangle. Bend your right knee and then slide your left foot about 6-12 inches in front of you. Line up your fingers with your pinky toe. Shift your body weight to the front foot and then lift the back leg up. Also, lift your arms straight up and gaze to the ceiling.

9. Parsvottanasana or Intense side stretch

This is a forward fold pose that promotes the downward and outward energy flow of the body. In this pose, one needs to surrender yourself into the depth of the pose. Alignment is a very important factor in order to be fully one with the Parsvottanasana. Doing this pose correctly calms the not only the mind but the body as well. Also, it helps tone leg, improve balance, and stretch your spine, hips, shoulders, and hamstrings.

How to do it:

The best way to start is by doing the mountain pose. Step one foot back approximately 4-5 feet away from the other and position it at a 45 degree angle. Ground both feet onto the mat. Lift your arms up and join the palms together at your upper back. Next, hinge forward and lengthen your spine. Lift your shoulders up, with palms together, as far as you can. Feel as your chest opens as you extend your arms up. Don't forget to breathe. Deepen your pose and hold it for several breaths.

10. Tree Pose

This pose tries to imitate the steady stature of a tree. It helps strengthen your thighs, legs, and back. The challenge however somehow increases since you have to hold this pose with only one leg on the ground. A distracted mind and poor attention may hinder a person from keeping balance and holding the pose for longer periods of time. In doing this pose, it is best to imagine yourself as a real tree with your foot as the root and your leg as the trunk. If you master this pose, you'll be likened to a tree that can maintain balance even with the presence of the wind.

How to do it:

To do the tree pose, start with doing the mountain pose. Bend one knee and use your hand to place your foot into the inner thigh. If you find this difficult, you can opt to place your foot to the shin below your knee. Remember not to position it on your knees. Lengthen up and shift your weight to your standing foot. Breathe normally and try to hold the pose as long as possible.

11. Dolphin Pose

Dolphin pose is an inversion and a forward bend pose. It is a variation of the downward facing dog wherein the forearms, instead of the palms, are on the ground. This pose helps strengthen the arms, shoulders, spine and abdominal muscles. It is very helpful in building upper body strength and is a good preparation for forearm stand and headstand.

How to do it:

Start on all of your fours with knees positioned beneath your hips and your wrists beneath your shoulders. Bring your elbows on the floor and make sure it is lined with your shoulders. Your forearms should also be parallel on the floor. Next, straighten your legs as if you were doing the downward facing dog. Allow your head to hang off the floor and look at your toes.

12. Plank

Plank is another foundational pose in yoga. It is an arm balancing pose that helps you strengthen your abdomen, spine, and arms. In this pose, you hold yourself as if you are a sturdy wooden plank. This pose allows you to gain the power that is required in doing other more complex poses. Plank is a part of the sun salutation series and is also used as a transition in doing different poses.

How to do it:

Use the downward facing dog as your starting position in doing the plank. Then, shift yourself forward so that your shoulders are stacked directly over your wrists. Lengthen the crown of your head forward while reaching your heels back. Make sure your hands are well grounded onto the mat. Spread your collarbones away from your sternum and lift your front body up. You are somehow doing a push up, but you extend your hands and straighten your body as much as possible. Hold the position for several breaths.

13. Side plank

The side plank is a great pose that helps build a strong core. It is also an arm-balance pose that helps strengthen your arms and wrist.

How to do it:

The first thing to do is lie on your left side with your knees straight. Place your forearm on your mat, under your shoulders, and make sure it is perpendicular to your body. Lift your body up until it forms a straight line. Place one foot on top of the other. Find your balance and hold the pose for several breaths.

14. Four-limbed staff pose or Chaturanga Dandasana

The Chaturanga is perhaps one of the most challenging pose in yoga and often times, it is performed incorrectly. There is a tendency to rush in doing the pose that most times the alignment is being taken for granted. If done incorrectly, it can hurt the joints of the shoulders. It is a major part of Vinyasa, Ashtanga, and Power Yoga that is why it is present in almost all sequence. This pose is a low plank and it will surely challenge you physically and mentally. This pose helps strengthen your arms, wrists, back, and abdomen. Also, it is a good preparation for more challenging arm balancing poses.

How to do it:

Use the plank pose as your starting position. Then, slowly bend your elbows to a 90 degree angle. Make sure that your arms are parallel to the floor. Spread your collarbones widely and ground your palms onto the mat. Next, slowly lift yourself away from the floor, pulling your front ribs into your spine. Also lift your upper thighs as you reach your tailbone towards your heels. Look forward and don't forget to breathe.

15. Bow

This pose is called this way since it resembles an archer's bow. The legs and the torso represent the bow's body while the arms act as the strings. The bow pose stimulates the reproductive organs and is a good stress reliever and fatigue buster. It also opens up the chest, shoulders, and neck and it strengthens both leg and arm muscles.

How to do it:

First step in doing this pose is to lie on your stomach with your feet hip-width apart. Place your arms on the sides, flat on the floor. Then, begin folding your knees and hold your ankles. While breathing in, lift your chest off the ground and pull your legs up. Look straight and hold the pose for as many breaths possible. Take long deep breaths and remember not to overdo the pose.

16. Bound angle pose

The bound angle is a famous seated yoga position that is good in opening the hips and groin. It is a very easy and relaxing pose that beginners would surely master. As a restorative pose, it calms and relaxes the mind, body and spirit.

How to do it:

Sit on the floor with your legs extended together straight in front of you. Bend your knees and join the soles of your feet together while remaining seated upright. Draw your feet as close to your body and gaze forward as you hold the pose for several breaths.

17. Camel Pose

The Camel pose is a powerful back bending pose that stretches your spine and back muscles. This pose will make you more flexible and it also helps improves digestion. This pose is best done after the other poses that involve much stretching and work.

How to do it:

Kneel with your knees and toes hip-distant apart. Your shoulders and knees should be in line and make sure your sole are facing the ceiling. Place your hands on your hips and get your balance. Then reach backward and grasp both your ankles while slowly lifting your chest up. Breathe and try to deepen your post by opening your chest even more. Keep in mind that your thighs should remain straight. If possible, perform the pose in front of a wall.

18. Bridge Pose

The bridge pose is a mild inversion pose that opens up your chest and shoulder area. This pose stimulates abdominal organs and glands which then improves digestion and metabolism. It helps you get relief from fatigue, stress, anxiety, and even depression because it is very effective in calming the mind.

How to do it:

Position to lie on your back. Make sure that both of your knees are bent with hip distance apart. Your feet should lay parallel and kept flat on the floor. Bring your arms under your thighs and try to clasp your hands together. Then, place your weight onto your feet and lift your hips up towards the ceiling. Roll your shoulder blades closer and try to hold the pose for as long as you can.

19. Wheel Pose

The wheel pose is a full backbend pose that demands flexibility and strength so it is best to learn camel and bridge pose before doing this. This pose strengthens and stretches the spine and back muscles. It opens up the chest and allows increased flow of oxygen to your lungs.

How to do it:

First, you have to lie flat on the floor. Bend your knees and bring the soles of your feet to your buttocks as close. Next, bend your arms and place your palms flat on the floor, right beside your ears with fingers facing your toes. Slowly lift your chest and hips off the floor, straighten your arms and lift your body through your shoulders. Hold the pose as long as you can and don't forget to breathe. To release the pose, bend your arms and slowly lower your upper back down to the floor.

20. Boat Pose

The boat is a great pose for strengthening the abdominal muscles. It is a very challenging pose as it requires you to have a strong core and good balance. This maybe a difficult pose at first, but as you practice and get better, it will give long lasting results.

How to do it:

Start this pose by sitting with your knees bent. Then, place your hands underneath your knees. Slightly bend back and slowly lift your shins parallel to the floor. Stretch your arms forward and straighten your knees if you can.

21. Seated Forward Fold

This pose is considered a very basic pose yet it poses a challenge especially to beginners. It is a great pose which strengthens the hamstrings and legs. Tt massages the internal organs and gives your spine a good stretch as well.

How to do it:

Sit on your mat with your legs together, extended in front of you and then point your toes straight to the ceiling. Sit straight up and make sure your spine is straight. Hinge forward and grab the sides of your feet. Bring yourself forward and try to bend your upper body as deep as you can and don't forget to continue breathing. Be careful not to fold your knees while doing this pose.

22. Crow Pose

This pose is also known as the crane or Bakasana pose. It is an arm balance which strengthens the wrists, arms, and abdominal muscles. This pose requires strength and balance that is why you should expect falling several times. But, once you gain mastery of the pose, it becomes fun and you will feel more confident and fulfilled about yourself.

How to do it:

First step for this pose is to do a deep squat with your knees wide apart and your feet together. Then place your hands on the floor and position it a bit wider than shoulder-width apart. Keep your palms flat on the floor as well. Next, position your knees at the back of your arms, on your triceps. Keep your feet together and slowly lift them up, with your weight concentrated on your arms. Find your balance as you lift your back and keep your gaze forward. For starters, you may be able to do this pose for a few seconds but don't worry, as you practice, you will surely find your balance.

23. Child's Pose

The child's pose is a forward bend and a relaxation pose that can be done in between asanas. It stretches your back and arms as you take a break from your sequence. Whenever you feel tired, you can always rest in your child's pose.

How to do it:

Start by kneeling down with your feet together. Position your buttocks toward your heels as you fold your body down and stretch forward. Rest your arms in a relaxed position, flat on the floor, and rest your stomach on top of your thighs. Bring your head down as well. You can close your eyes to get a more relaxing feeling.

24. Handstand

The handstand is one of the more challenging yoga inversion poses. This pose decompresses the spine and strengthens the arms, shoulders, and wrists. It is also a great pose to improve balance and focus. This pose requires preparation that is why first timers may not perform this pose right away. However, one can always perform this pose with assistance from another or from a wall.

How to do it:

Do the downward facing dog as your starting position. Place your hands approximately a foot away from the wall and then move one foot forward while lifting the other leg into the air. Bend your knee and hop the other foot to bring both feet up to the wall. After which, join your legs together and extend your heels up to the ceiling.

25. Headstand

The headstand is often considered the king of yoga poses because of the many benefits it can give you. It increases blood and nutrient flow in your body and it also strengthen the muscles of the body.

How to do it:

Begin by doing the child's pose. Relax and monitor your breathing for a few moments. Then, lift your head and move your elbows to the ground a feet or two in front of your knees. Wrap your hands around each elbow without lifting them up. Plant your elbows and ground yourself onto the mat. Release your hands and interlace them in front without moving your elbows. Slowly lift your heads up and position your head into the palm of your hands. Walk your feet towards your face and lift them naturally as you shift your weight to your elbows. Straighten your legs and hold it as long as you can. You can have someone assist you or you perform this pose with a wall in front.

26. Shoulder stand

If the headstand is the king of all yoga poses, the shoulder stand is the queen. It is an inversion that provides a lot of great benefits. The thing is it is more accessible than the other inversions such as headstand and handstand. However, this maybe a dangerous pose especially with the neck that is why one needs to be careful in performing shoulder stand.

How to do it:

The first thing to do is to lie down on your back. Place your arms right beside you and make yourself comfortable. Then, lift your legs straight up towards the ceiling. Slowly lift your hips off the floor and support them by placing your hands at the upper back. Continue lifting yourself up until you are able to straighten your spine. Rest your weight on the back side of your shoulders, and not on your neck. Breathe and hold the pose as much as you can. To release the pose, bring one foot one at a time and release your arms afterwards.

27. Savasana or Corpse Pose

The Savasana is a relaxation pose that is done in between or after the asanas. It may seem to be a very simple pose but it requires a lot of concentration to perform. If done correctly, this pose stimulates blood and oxygen circulation and helps relieve stress and fatigue. At the end of each practice, this pose helps you absorb all the benefits of your practice.

How to do it:

To do this pose, lie flat on your mat. Separate your legs and feet apart while you place your arms comfortably at the sides facing up. Give yourself a little stretching until you become comfortable laying down. Then, close your eyes and breathe normally. Relax and allow your mind to calm down as you hold the pose for several minutes.

Chapter 4 - Breathing and Mediation

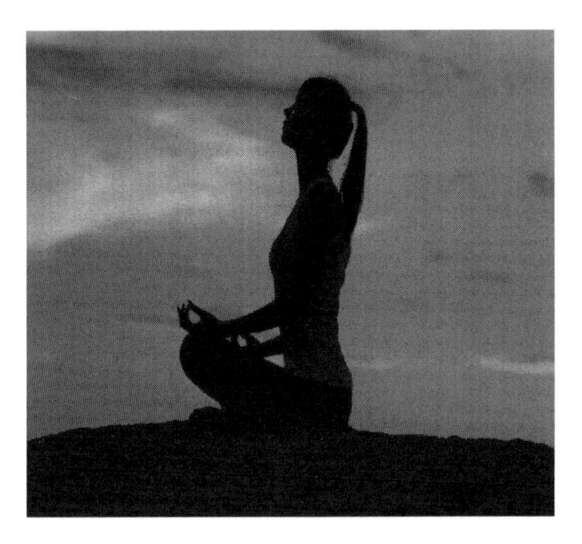

Aside from the poses, stretches, and physical exercises linked with yoga, meditation and breathing are the other two important components of the practice. The Pranayama, or yoga breathing and meditation, is considered very essential in the holistic development of a person's physical, mental, spiritual, and emotional well-being. The ultimate purpose of breathing and meditation is to give a person a sense of peace and calmness. It trains the mind and body to focus, slow down, maintain silence and be positive.

During the ancient times, the Pranayama was developed by yogis as a means of purification. The word is derived from "Prana" which means "life force energy", and "Yama" which translates to "mastery or control". Thus, the word Pranayama is simply to control, master, and change the life forces and energy of the body. If you feel stressed and you want to manage your anger and anxiety, making meditation as a part of your daily routine will surely be very helpful. It will make you feel more grounded and stable when so many things are starting to pull you in different directions.

In order to properly practice the art of breathing and meditation, it is important to learn the basics. Building a strong foundation is necessary for one to establish the proper breathing exercise.

With this, one must learn that the science of breath starts and ends with awareness. Yes, breath awareness is one key factor in order to build a strong connection between one's mind and body. One should develop the attitude of being curious of what is happening within and noticing how the breath operates. You have to feel the air go in and out of your nostrils, the diaphragm, and through your body as a whole.

Once you have already learned on focusing on your breathing, the next thing you need is to unlearn the tendency to control it. The art of allowing your breath is letting the breath happen instead of making it happen. This is also vital in the practice of correct breathing and meditation. Allowing your breath to flow prepares your mind to flow freely as well, which in turn will give you a sense of freedom.

Also, in order to build a good foundation with genuine interest, one must work around with the different irregularities that may affect breathing. These irregularities are mostly caused by the mind and to be aware, one must eliminate these distractions. The pauses, jerks, noise, and shallowness are among the most common breath irregularities. If you are able to remove these things from your physical breath, you will enjoy the benefits it has on the mind as well. You will experience more peace if your breathing comes in smooth, quiet, slow, and continuous.

Beginners in yoga tend to approach breathing and meditation separately from the physical practice. But, as one goes deeper into the practice of yoga, it must then be understood that breathing, meditation, and the physical components should work altogether. When you are able to control your mind and be in a state away from distraction and turbulence, contentment and happiness will arise from within. This feeling will then help you get though the everyday stressors you encounter.

To start off your breathing and meditation endeavor, here is a simple exercise to help you focus on your breathing. Follow these steps as you try to be in one with your breath.

1. Find a comfortable place wherein you can stay for a few minutes.
2. If possible, stay away from noise or distractions. You can stay in a room, or if you have the chance to, you can stay by the beach or someplace away from many people.
3. Sit comfortably, close your eyes and try to focus on your breathing
4. As you inhale, feel your ribs expand and your lungs inflate. Also, feel the air as it passes through your nostrils.
5. As you exhale, think about your lungs deflating and feel as the air rushes out of your nostrils.

6. At first, your mind will surely wander. Just try to turn your attention back to your breath if this occurs.
7. Repeat these steps for several minutes until you become comfortable with what you are doing. After some time, you will realize that it will come in naturally.

For a more advanced deep breathing meditation, you can practice by following the steps below. Deep breathing requires you to get as much air in and out of your lungs as you breathe deeply from the abdomen. Taking breaths from the abdomen allows you to inhale more oxygen which makes you less tense and anxious.

1. Find a comfortable place to stay and sit with your back straight. Then, place one hand on your

stomach and the other on your chest.

2. Breathe in through your nose and as you do this, the hand on your stomach should rise. On the other hand, the hand on your chest should only move a little.
3. Exhale through your mouth and as you do, push out as much air as you can while your abdomen contracts. This time, the hand on your stomach should move in while the other should still move a little.
4. Continue breathing in through your nose and breathing out your mouth. At first, you may find this exercise difficult as you will constantly watch your breathing but as you practice more and more, you will see that it will all come natural.

If at first, you will really find difficulty in doing this exercise while sitting down, you can try lying up on the floor. Instead of using your hands, you can place a small book on top of your stomach. Breathe in and out and feel as the book rises and falls.

Breathing in Asanas

While performing yoga poses or asanas, breathing is a very important thing to remember. In yoga, we want to achieve a calm mind and proper breathing is essential in order to do this. We have this tendency to hold our breath or engage in stress breathing especially when we perform challenging poses. This stresses and creates tension in the body. This is the reason why we need to watch our breathing and practice it together with the poses.

There are several ways to breathe during and in between asanas. There are different techniques that are suited to different postures and it is also important to know which ones to appropriately use.

The general rule in breathing is to breathe out for forward bends and breathe in for backward bends and stretches. You inhale to lengthen or open and exhale as you twist or relax. Some poses may also require you to hold your breath as well. Another technique used in most yoga postures is the Dirga Pranayama. For backbends and chest opening poses such as pigeon, bridge, warrior, one needs to focus on actively breathing. For forward folding and belly down poses such as child, boat and cobra, one needs to focus on breathing into the belly.

In order to increase focus and endurance for strength building postures, use the Ujjiaj Pranayama technique. This is also called the ocean sounding breath since you mimic the sound of the ocean by contracting the glottis with the inhalation and exhalation. To do this, you need to whisper the letter "h" while feeling the contraction in your throat. After several breaths, close your mouth and breathe through your noise while still making the ocean sound. If you want to get intense in holding a pose, you can use the Kapalabhati Pranayama. It is characterized by a passive inhalation and an active exhalation. To exhale, quickly pump air through your nose as if you are blowing a candle.

Getting used to the proper breathing patterns may take some time. Each person breathes differently and has varied pace. Don't worry if it takes you some time to find the right pace for your practice, just remember to keep breathing.

Chapter 5 - Yoga for a Better and Happier Life

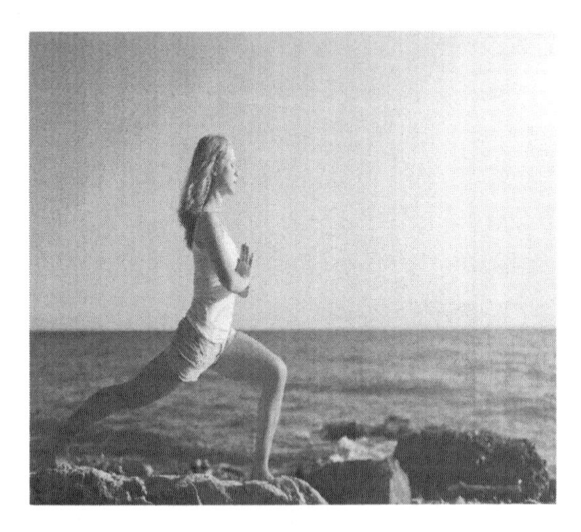

The best things about yoga are its benefits to a person's mind, body and even spiritual well-being. For several years, it has been proven to help manage stress and anxiety. Also, it gives the yogi a more positive outlook in life. Remember that yoga is not just about exercise, but it is about a healthy lifestyle. It gives a person the sense of peace, happiness, and tranquility.

One major benefit of yoga is that it strengthens your body and improves flexibility. After doing your first few sessions, you might feel sore and tired. You might not be able to fully perform the poses right away. But, as you continue your practice, you will see that you can slowly do the things you thought of was impossible. You will notice that it will get easier to carry your body and that your core, together with other muscles become strong each time.

Yoga also helps in maintaining a good posture and balance. As you become more flexible and strong, your posture develops as well. A lot of poses require you to stand or sit straight in order to get the full benefits of each one. As mentioned several times, yoga involves awareness and this helps you notice if you are slumping or slouching.

Doing yoga also leads to an increase blood flow and stronger immunity. Regular practice is also good for your heart. It has long been known that it can help slow the heart rate and lower blood pressure and cholesterol levels. Several yoga poses, including the inversions and some relaxation poses, help oxygen and nutrient circulation. When you do stretching and movements, you can also increase the activity in the lymphatic system. This helps you fight infection, dispose toxins, and destroy bad cells in the body.

Weight loss is also another benefit brought about by the practice of yoga. Performing the different poses requires a lot of muscle strength and as you hold each pose, you will surely burn some calories and shed some sweat. Some sequences and types of practice require vigorous movements that help yogis lose more. Also, yoga is an effective stress management strategy which then relates to the reduced likelihood of unhealthy stress eating. When paired with the right diet, yoga can indeed be a very good exercise for your weight loss goals.

As mentioned a lot of times, yoga helps you gain focus and attention. It allows you to be aware of yourself and your body. A lot of studies done have also shown that it improves IQ, memory, helps you solve problems and recall things easily. When you try to relax and slow down, your system shifts to a more calm and restorative state as well.

Being away from all distractions, both internal and external, gives you peace of mind. When you are away from anger, stress, fear, frustrations, and other negative energies, you have the opportunity to better connect with yourself as you do meditation and practice. Serotonin levels also increase which heightens the activity of some brain parts giving you greater feelings of happiness.

An increase in self-esteem is also seen in yogis who religiously practice. When you practice, you should have the intention to examine yourself and improve not only your physical self but also your mindset. Going deeper into practice allows you to experience empathy, forgiveness, and gratitude. It also allows you to feel that you are indeed part of something bigger in this life. Yoga provides you the needed tools to change in order to achieve a better life. You will see that yoga encourages you to better take care of yourself and others because it holds the belief that service is a way to give life meaning.

Chapter 6 - Additional Tips and Reminders

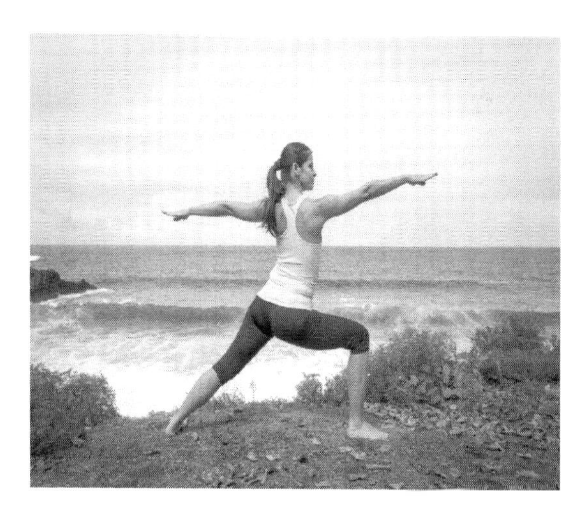

As a beginner you may find it intimidating to start a yoga practice. You may feel that a lot of things are holding you back and the thought of having to learn so many things might scare you. Here are a few tips and reminders to help you if you decide to start a new journey in yoga.

1. **Keep a journal**
   Every day is a new experience in yoga. Your teacher might give you

several comments and you yourself might discover a lot of things as you engage in practice. It is best to record your insights and thoughts in a journal to somehow see the progress you are making each time.

2. **Turn off your gadgets**
   In yoga, you need to focus your attention to your body that is why bringing gadgets with you during practice might be a bad idea. You need to get away from unnecessary distraction that is why you definitely need to turn all those gadgets off.

3. **Never compare yourself with others**
   Each one starts as a beginner and remember that one person is different from the other. Some people might be naturally flexible, some might be a bit stronger than you are and there is nothing wrong

with that. The mistake comes in when you start to compare yourself with what others can and cannot do. It will only lead to jealousy and frustrations during practice.

4. **Do not be afraid to rest**
   Whether you are in a one on one or group class, never be ashamed to take rests in between poses. If you feel tired from performing challenging asanas, you can always rest in your child's pose or in Savasana. There is no competition in the practice of yoga and you do not need to be a show off. If your body cannot perform any more poses, then take a short break.

5. **Be familiar with the names of poses**
   During practice, instructors will give out the name of the poses and then show you how to do it. If you have an idea what the pose is, you

wouldn't have to keep looking at how the instructor does it. It will save you and your neck the energy from looking around. Be familiar with the positions and if possible know the steps before going into class.

6. **Avoid going to practice with a full stomach**
   It is recommended for you to have an empty stomach 2-3 hours before practice. This will help you feel lighter so that you can move easily. Also, this will prevent you from feeling uncomfortable especially when doing bends and inversions.

7. **Smile**
   Smiling helps relax the body and mind. It gives you a more positive mindset and with it, you will surely enjoy your practice even more.

8. Thank yourself after every practice

After you've done your first class, and all the other succeeding ones, always remember to thank yourself. Thank your body for doing a great job. Yoga is not an easy practice and the mere fact that you have decided to start on a new journey should already give you the feeling of satisfaction and fulfillment.

CONCLUSION

Now you have reached the last part of this book. Thank you again for downloading this book!

I hope this book was able to help you get to know what yoga is, how it is done, and how its benefits can help you become a better individual.

The next step upon successful completion of this book is to get yourself all the things you need and start doing your own practice. Find a class or an instructor who can help you achieve your goals. There is no need to worry about anything. Do not wait any longer and start a new journey towards a happier and healthier life with yoga.

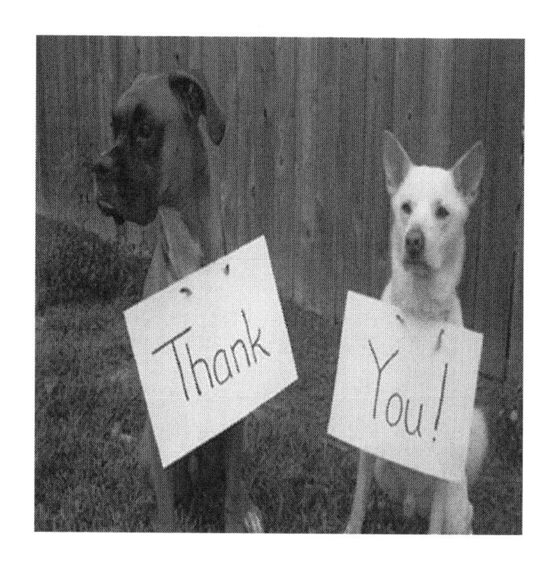

Finally, if you enjoyed this book, then I'd like to ask you for a favor, would you be kind enough to leave a review for this book on Amazon? It'd be greatly appreciated!

Click here to leave a review for this book on Amazon!

Thank you and good luck!

13875160R00048

Printed in Great Britain
by Amazon.co.uk, Ltd.,
Marston Gate.